THE
GASTROPARESIS
COOKBOOK
FOR TWO

50 delicious & easy to prepare
recipes to help manage
gastroparesis

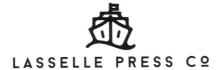

LASSELLE PRESS CO

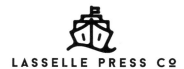

LASSELLE PRESS C⚬

ISBN-13: 978-1911364962
ISBN-10: 1911364960

CONTENTS

CHAPTER 7
VEGETARIAN
ENTRÉES | 49

CHAPTER 8
STOCKS & SAUCES | 61

CHAPTER 9
DRINKS & DESSERTS | 71

CONVERSION TABLES | 77

BIBLIOGRAPHY | 79

INDEX | 80

INTRODUCTION

Welcome to The Gastroparesis Cookbook For Two.

A diagnosis of gastroparesis can be a daunting time, both for you and your partner. Equally, if your partner is suffering from the symptoms of this condition, then it is likely that you want to do all that you can to help.

As you probably already know, gastroparesis is a chronic condition that can be extremely difficult to live with. However, with the right treatments, foods and professional guidance, you can start to feel better again.

This cookbook has been created to give you and your partner an overview of gastroparesis; the symptoms and possible causes; the foods you should be limiting or avoiding; and the ones you can continue to eat. As well as this, we outline the minerals and nutrient consumption that you will need to manage such as fiber, fat and carbohydrates. The guidance provided in this book should always go along with that of your doctor or dietitian's recommendations.

Lastly, we provide over 50 recipes specifically created for two people so that you can continue to enjoy cooking and eating together, regardless of whether one or both of you is suffering from gastroparesis. Each recipe has its nutritional information broken down so that you can easily plan your daily or weekly meals.

Our aim is to help you enjoy life in the best possible way by eating foods that will minimize your symptoms and taste delicious, using easy to find ingredients and simple instructions.

We wish you all the best on your journey to wellness.

Happy cooking!

The Lasselle Press Team

I

UNDERSTANDING GASTROPARESIS

Whether you have already been diagnosed with gastroparesis, or you've been experiencing uncomfortable symptoms that you think could be gastroparesis, this chapter aims to help by providing information about the condition. Hopefully, it will give you a little more confidence to seek medical advice from your doctor if you haven't already done so. And if you've been diagnosed already, then we hope that this book can provide you with a little more insight and confidence in your decisions about what to eat.

GASTROPARESIS:

Gastroparesis affects the stomach and the digestive system. When suffering from the condition, your stomach will be less able to digest foods as well as it should do. This can affect your nutrient intake, both due to the problems with the digestion system and because of under-eating/ not being able to consume the same variety of food you may be used to. Unfortunately, gastroparesis usually leads to uncomfortable symptoms in sufferers, especially after eating.

To explain the condition further you will need to know a little more about the stomach: the stomach muscles usually work to contract and digest food before passing this digested food through to the intestines, and ultimately out of the body. Both solids and liquids are processed in this way and are broken down into tiny particles. Thus, liquids and soft foods are always easier to digest than solids as they start as smaller particles to begin with.

For those suffering with gastroparesis, the stomach muscles do not work in the way that they should do, which is usually caused by damage to the vagus nerve. This nerve is responsible for controlling the stomach muscles' movements and contractions. As a result of poor muscle movement and slow digestion, the food is not broken down as it should be. This delays the stomach from emptying and so food can remain there for long periods of time, and in some cases, stay there. This can lead to further problems such as bacteria growth in the stomach and bezoars.

CAUSES OF GASTROPARESIS:

There are a variety of potential causes of gastroparesis. In certain individuals, the cause is unknown (idiopathic) and cannot be pinned down to any one factor. However, other possible causes are outlined below:

DIABETES TYPE 1 AND TYPE 2: If uncontrolled and sugar levels are not regulated, this can lead to gastroparesis.

ABDOMINAL SURGERY THAT INJURES THE VAGUS NERVE: Often a complication of gastric bypass surgery.

CERTAIN MEDICATIONS: Including certain tricyclic antidepressants, calcium channel blockers and narcotics, nicotine, progesterone, lithium and clonidine (always speak to your doctor if unsure).

HORMONAL DISORDERS (ENDOCRINE): Addison's disease, hyperparathyroidism, hypothyroidism, or hormone imbalance. Consult your doctor if you have any of these and notice the symptoms outlined in the next chapter.

AUTOIMMUNE DISEASES: Parkinson's, multiple sclerosis and others (controlling inflammation is really important here). Consult your doctor if you have any of these and notice the symptoms outlined in the next chapter.

EATING DISORDERS: Anorexia and Bulimia. It is important to consider that you may suffer from gastroparesis if you are suffering, or have suffered, one of these disorders. Again, consult your doctor if you experience any unusual symptoms.

SYMPTOMS:

The following symptoms may be an indicator of gastroparesis. Please consult your doctor to discuss these symptoms:

- Heartburn,
- Nausea,
- Stomach pain,
- Vomiting undigested food,
- Feeling full very quickly after eating,
- Bloating of the abdominal cavity,
- Weight loss and a loss of appetite,
- Fluctuating blood sugar levels - particularly problematic for those with diabetes,
- Bacteria growth on the stomach lining, leading to bacterial infections in the body (this would need to be diagnosed by a professional).

These symptoms may not necessarily indicate gastroparesis and may be symptoms of other illnesses or diseases, so you should always consult a professional for a diagnosis. Likewise, it could be that these symptoms are a result of gastroparesis as well as another disease or illness. If you're suffering from a known disease but notice these symptoms, or anything out of the ordinary, you must see your doctor.

TREATING GASTROPARESIS:

Eating a healthy and controlled diet can help control the symptoms of gastroparesis but cannot cure or treat it alone. It is crucial that a healthcare professional diagnose this condition and offer support and medication as well as dietary and lifestyle advice; there are also procedures that can help with emptying the stomach. This book should be used as a guide alongside this information and aims to provide you with recommended dietary choices as well as recipes to try out in the kitchen. It is also important to take into consideration, any other dietary restrictions you may have as a result of other conditions including diabetes, celiac disease, or lactose intolerance.

Alongside your diet, you may find that changes to your lifestyle will have a positive impact on your symptoms. Consider the following:

1. Exercise: it is recommended that you exercise for at least 20-30 minutes per day. This can be either a walk, jog, yoga, or even something a little more strenuous.
2. Drink plenty of water: this will not only keep you hydrated but will aid the digestive system.
3. Sleep: try and get 8 hours sleep per night.
4. Posture: sit upright as much as you can, in particular when relaxing. It is important to find a chair that will help with this posture in order to help the digestive system. After meals, stay sitting upright or try to go for a light walk.

II

DIET AND NUTRITION TIPS FOR GASTROPARESIS

RECOMMENDATIONS FOR THE GASTROPARESIS DIET:

- Liquids are easier to digest than solids so make the most of wholesome broths and soups as well as shakes, particularly when your symptoms flare up.
- Eating little and often is far better than eating big portions. Aim for 5-6 small meals a day rather than 3 big ones.
- Aim to consume less than 40g fat per day. If you're eating 6 meals per day then your fat intake should be 6-7g per meal.
- Thoroughly chew each mouthful to give your stomach a hand! Soft, ground, strained or puréed foods are easier to digest than solids.
- FODMAPS - consider restricting FODMAPS (more information in the next section).
- Avoid red meat.
- Eat and drink separately.
- Lower your fiber intake - especially whole grains, raw fruit and vegetables with skins, and wheat.
- Avoid foods high in fructose and polyols (artificial sweeteners like sorbitol).
- Take a walk or ensure you sit upright after eating (for at least one hour) in order to aid the digestion process.
- Peel fruit and vegetables before blending, cooking or straining.
- Low fat dairy options are advised - some milk products may flare up symptoms, so it is important that you monitor your reactions to these and choose dairy-free alternatives if lactose intolerant.
- Given that you are going to need to lower your fat, fiber and sugar intake, it can sometimes be difficult to meet your daily nutritional needs. Speak to your doctor or dietitian about supplementing your diet with multivitamins such as B6, B12, fish oils etc. This will depend on the vitamins you are lacking from the foods you are reducing or avoiding. Other than multivitamins, shakes and smoothies are a great way of consuming vitamins.

OTHER DIETARY CONSIDERATIONS

FODMAPS (Fermentable Oligosaccharides, Disaccharides, Monosaccharides and Polyols)

These are simple and complex sugars that are poorly absorbed after food has been digested. They are found in a variety of fruits, vegetables, milk, and wheat. They pass through the stomach and the small intestine without changing state and are then fermented by colonic bacteria, resulting in a release of gas; or they are expelled from the body with fluids. The retention of these sugars often leads to bloating, abdominal pain and diarrhoea, particularly for those with sensitive stomachs and IBS. For some with gastroparesis, FODMAPS can make digestion even harder. Please note that your reaction to these types of foods vary between patients, and these are suggestions to the types of foods you could consider monitoring.

FODMAP foods to avoid include:
* Onion, garlic, pulses, brassicas (cauliflower, broccoli, cabbage etc.),
* Wheat,
* Fruit e.g. plums, peaches, nectarines, apples and other stoned fruits,
* Lactose (for those who are lactose intolerant).

Diabetes

If you have diabetes and gastroparesis, this can be extremely confusing and difficult to manage. The major consideration here is controlling your blood sugar levels. This can be done through insulin as well as your diet. Meals should be kept small and eaten at regular times. You should continue to eat carbohydrates in equal proportions for each meal to help regulate your blood sugar levels. It is recommended that you consume between 30-40g carbohydrates per meal and eat 6 meals per day. You should be consuming between 210-240g carbohydrates per day depending on your gender and size and what your doctor has recommended. Speak to a professional if unsure.

Gluten-Free

For some, going gluten-free can help control symptoms of gastroparesis. For those suffering from celiac disease or gluten allergies this is essential.

Dairy-Free

Lactose in dairy products can flare up symptoms for some, and if you're lactose intolerant, need avoiding. In this case, just substitute any dairy items in the recipes with dairy free. We've included a great almond milk and rice milk recipe to use too!

GERD friendly

Gastroesophageal reflux disease can cause uncomfortable symptoms such as heartburn and is caused by different foods which range from one person to another. Common foods that flare symptoms are tomatoes, citrus, spices and chocolate.

FOODS TO ADD TO YOUR SHOPPING LIST:

Ginger ale
Fat-free soups
Bouillon soups
Saltine crackers
Skim milk
Skim milk products
Low-fat Greek yogurt
Low-fat cheese
Fat free soups
Fat-free broths
Vegetable soups
White bread, rice or pasta
Eggs (limit egg yolks)
Peanut butter (up to 2 tbsp per day)
Vegetable juices
Beets
Carrots
Mushrooms
Spinach
Summer squash
Acorn squash
Strained tomato sauce
Yams
Apple juice
Grape juice
Pineapple juice
Cranberry juice
Coconut oil
Frozen yogurt
Gelatin
Jelly
Skinless chicken and turkey breasts
Ground lean chicken and turkey
Soft fish e.g. sea bass, cod, haddock
Apple sauce
Skinless peaches and pears

Sparkling water
Margarines and butters (in small amounts)
Low-fat mayonnaise
Gluten free foods
Gluten free pasta and bread
White bread
Canned fruits (skinless)
Extra virgin olive oil
Egg noodles
Rice cakes
Honey
Maple syrup
Green tea
Tea
Gatorade

Stock your pantry with:
Dried herbs: thyme, basil, sage, tarragon, parsley etc.
Dried spices: cinnamon, ground nutmeg, ground ginger, cloves

FOODS TO AVOID:

Whole milk products
Creams
Soups that are made with cream or whole milk
Fatty broths
Fruits with skin on and dried fruits
Steak and red meat
Peas
Dried beans
Lentils
Oatmeal
Cereal
Whole grain rice
Whole grain bread
Raw vegetables
Green beans, wax, and Lima beans with skins
Brussels spouts
Cauliflower
Corn
Cabbage
Celery

Onion
Peppers
Eggplant
Turnips
Sauerkraut
Water chestnuts
Desserts high in fat, such as cakes, cookies, ice cream, pies, or pastries
Fruit preservatives
Packaged and processed foods
Cayenne pepper

III

EATING OUT AND SHOPPING GUIDE

After receiving a diagnosis of gastroparesis, or even before, you may have found the idea or experience of eating out quite intimidating. Just one look at the menu and all those rich, fatty food options probably send your mind straight to the thought of pain and flare ups. It can be an uncomfortable, if not distressing time, but having gastroparesis needn't mean you can't enjoy eating out with friends and family.

TIPS FOR EATING OUT:

- Suggest a restaurant to friends and family once you've browsed their menu and made sure that there is at least one dish on there that would be suitable for you to order.
- Consider calling the restaurant beforehand to explain the types of foods you can and can't have. Those working in this industry will usually be more than happy to cater for specific dietary needs and if they're not, they're not worth your custom!
- Ask for dishes to be cooked in olive oil rather than butter or vegetable oils.
- Opt for seafood or poultry options and ask how they're cooked.
- Drink before or after your meal and not during.
- Ask about small or half portions and order these.
- Don't let yourself go hungry before you go out; work out if this is going to be the last meal of the day and if so have your other meals beforehand. If it's lunchtime, ensure you have eaten enough meals beforehand and that you will be able to eat the rest of your meals afterwards.

GROCERY SHOPPING:

1. Always write a list and check it against the recommended foods as well as those that are not allowed.
2. Plan out your meals so that you know exactly how much of each item you need.
3. Check out the reduced items section to see what bargains you can get your hands on!
4. Ask your family to support you and try similar foods to you, so that you don't have temptations lying around the kitchen. Obviously they will need to eat a different diet to you and bigger portions, but they could try and stick to foods such as poultry and seafood instead of red meats and fatty foods.
5. Don't grocery shop on an empty stomach - you'll only find yourself tempted by snacks and convenient foods.

TRAVELING:

It may be difficult to go out for the whole day, let alone the weekend, week, or even longer! The thought of not having foods available to you can be daunting; you really wouldn't want to find yourself in the position of grabbing something from the shop or café, just because you're hungry and in a rush.

Prep your meals for the day and store them in containers. If you're not going to be somewhere with a microwave, ensure these can be eaten cold and straight from the container. If you're staying away, you could always take extra portions for the next day and ask the hotel to store them for you and even heat them up.

It's also worth researching the restaurants and cafés where you are visiting and following the advice given for eating out. Creating a meal plan for the duration of your stay is a good idea, so that you are not left in a tricky situation. Finally, taking pre-made shakes and smoothies is a great way to consume your calories whilst on the move.

EATING FOR TWO:

While it is unlikely that both you and your partner suffer from gastroparesis, it is always easier to stick to a new diet or regime if you have support. These recipes have been created for two people. If your partner does not suffer from gastroparesis, they should eat bigger portions and more variety. However you can simply multiply the serving size, making it easier for you to stick to your serving size of the right foods as well as not having to cook up two separate meals. Your partner could then add a side of fruit or vegetables to boost their nutrients and vitamins. As always, please consult your doctor before making any changes to your diet and ask about any vitamin supplements you may need.

IV
GETTING STARTED

KITCHEN EQUIPMENT:

In order to help you get started on this diet, there are a few things that you will need to be able to prepare the foods and meals in this cookbook:

- Blender/ food processor
- Crock pot, pots, skillet
- Steam basket/steamer/colander
- Oven dish, tray
- Potato masher
- Large mixing bowls
- Foil/plastic wrap
- Tupperware boxes
- Stocking your cupboard:
- Ensure you purchase a variety of dry ingredients that can be used to add flavor to your foods (see foods to enjoy list).

KEEPING A FOOD JOURNAL:

It is always a good idea to keep a record of the foods and drinks you consume as well as your symptoms. This way you can track when your symptoms flare up and what may have caused them to do so. In the same way, if you're working to cut out a certain food group at a time, this is a great method for seeing if it makes a difference, as well as if there are certain foods that you know you should avoid. Like any condition, each person experiences gastroparesis differently, and while some foods will be okay for one person, they may be intolerable for others. Keep a journal and use this alongside your doctor's recommendations and these recipes, to work out what's best for you.

Now that you have all you need to know to get your kitchen stocked with the right foods and equipment; you've planned out how many meals you need a day; and you know what you can eat - you're ready to go! The gastroparesis road can be long and taxing but hopefully with the following recipes and a lot of self-love and encouragement, you will be able to control your symptoms as best as possible, continue to enjoy meal times, and feel happier and healthier again.

We wish you all the luck and support on this journey.

BREAKFAST

BANANA PANCAKES

SERVES 2 / PREP TIME: 5 MINUTES / COOK TIME: 5 MINUTES

Pancakes work wonders for one of your small meals a day.

---

1 VERY RIPE SMALL BANANA

2 LARGE EGG WHITES

1/2 CUP NON-FAT GREEK YOGURT

---

1. Blend all the ingredients in a food processor until smooth.
2. Heat a non-stick skillet over a medium heat.
3. Pour batter into pancake shapes and cook for 1-2 minutes on each side.
4. Enjoy!

Per serving: Calories: 133; Fat:0g (Saturated Fat: 0g); Carbohydrates: 17g; Fiber: 1g; Sugar: 11g; Sodium: 164mg; Protein: 17g; Potassium 422mg

SPICED PUMPKIN PANCAKES

SERVES 2 / PREP TIME: 3 MINUTES / COOK TIME: 10 MINUTES

Deliciously spiced cinnamon and pumpkin breakfast treat.

1/4 CUP SOLID PACK PUMPKIN (ORGANIC PREFERABLY)

2 LARGE EGG WHITES

1/2 TSP CINNAMON

1 TSP OLIVE OIL

---

1. Blend pumpkin in a food processor until completely puréed.
2. Whisk together the egg whites, cinnamon and puréed pumpkin in a mixing bowl.
3. Heat the olive oil in a pan over a medium heat.
4. Pour 1/2 the batter into the pan and cook for 4-5 minutes.
5. Flip over and cook the other side for 1-2 minutes.
6. Repeat for the second pancake.
7. Serve with your choice of sweet accompaniment (honey or maple syrup) or alone for a savory breakfast.

Per serving: Calories: 68; Fat: 5g (Saturated Fat: 1g); Carbohydrates: 3g; Fiber: 1g; Sugar: 1; Sodium: 154mg; Protein: 4g; Potassium: 119mg

TURKEY BROTH

SERVES 2 / PREP TIME: 5 MINUTES / COOK TIME: 30 MINUTES

Can be enjoyed for a warming breakfast or throughout the day.

4OZ SKINLESS, BONELESS TURKEY BREAST (WHOLE IF POSSIBLE)

1/2 CUP LOW SODIUM CHICKEN STOCK

1 CUP WATER

1/4 CUP ACORN SQUASH, PEELED AND CHOPPED

1 TSP DRIED THYME

1 TSP DRIED SAGE

---

1. Bring a large pot of water to the boil over a high heat.
2. Add the turkey breast meat and poach in the water over a medium heat for 10-15 minutes or until cooked throughout and not pink.
3. Meanwhile, cook your squash by steaming over the pot for the same amount of time as the turkey (make sure these are extremely soft).
4. Remove the turkey and squash once cooked.
5. Slice the turkey breast.
6. Into a new pan add all of the ingredients and bring to the boil over a high heat.
7. Lower the heat and allow to simmer for 10-15 minutes.
8. Serve right away!

Hint: If you need to puree your vegetables, simply blend the whole broth in a food processor until completely smooth.

Per serving: Calories: 79; Fat: 2g (Saturated Fat: 0g); Carbohydrates: 3g; Fiber: 1g; Sugar: 0; Sodium: 43mg; Protein: 14g; Potassium: 262mg

BERRY & CREAM OF WHEAT BREAKFAST

SERVES 2 / PREP TIME: 2 MINUTES / COOK TIME: 10 MINUTES

Tart and tasty!

1 CUP SKIM MILK	**1/4 CUP CANNED RASPBERRIES (SKINLESS)**
1 CUP WATER	**1 TSP SUGAR**
1/4 CUP CREAM OF WHEAT	**1 TSP GROUND NUTMEG**

1. Bring the milk and water to the boil in a pot and reduce to a simmer.
2. Stir in the cream of wheat until the sauce starts to thicken (over a low heat).
3. Leave to simmer for 2-3 minutes, then stir in the berries.
4. Serve with the nutmeg and sugar sprinkled over the top.

Hint: Skip the sugar if you're diabetic - the berries should be sweet enough!

Per serving: Calories: 142; Fat: 1g (Saturated Fat: 0g); Carbohydrates: 27g; Fiber: 2g; Sugar: 10g; Sodium: 61mg; Protein: 7g; Potassium: 247mg

VITAMIN BREAKFAST SMOOTHIE

SERVES 2 / PREP TIME: 5 MINUTES / COOK TIME: NA

Pack a tall glass with these healthy ingredients and enjoy a sweet start to your day!

1/2 CUP NON-FAT GREEK YOGURT

1/2 SMALL PEELED BANANA, FRESH OR FROZEN

1/4 CUP CANNED BLUEBERRIES, SKIN-LESS& UNSWEETENED

1 TBSP SMOOTH PEANUT BUTTER

1/2 TSP CINNAMON

---

1. Blend all ingredients in a smoothie maker until there are no lumps left.
2. Serve over crushed ice!
3. Sprinkle a little more cinnamon over the top if desired.

Hint: If you need to, strain the smoothie through a muslin cloth or sieve to get rid of any little bits that may be left from the fruit.

Per serving: Calories: 142; Fat: 5g (Saturated Fat: 1g); Carbohydrates: 19g; Fiber: 2g; Sugar: 11g; Sodium: 58mg; Protein: 9g; Potassium; 353mg

CHIVE & BEET FRITTATA

SERVES 2 / PREP TIME: 5 MINUTES / COOK TIME: 10 MINUTES

This is a fast and fresh breakfast that can be cooked up in advance.

---

3 EGG WHITES

2 TBSP CHOPPED CHIVES

1 TSP DRIED BASIL

1 TBSP NON-FAT GREEK YOGURT

1 TSP OLIVE OIL

1/4 CUP CANNED BEETS, SLICED

---

1. Preheat the broiler/grill on a low heat.
2. Whisk the eggs, chives, basil and Greek yogurt together.
3. Pour the mixture into a lightly oiled shallow baking dish/oven-proof skillet.
4. Layer the top of the frittata with the sliced beets.
5. Place under the broiler for 6-8 minutes or until cooked through.
6. Slice and serve!

Hint: If you want to make this ahead of time, simply follow the above instructions, allow to cool and then wrap in foil and refrigerate for up to 2 days.

Per serving: Calories: 57; Fat: 2g (Saturated Fat: 0g); Carbohydrates: 3g; Fiber: 1g; Sugar: 2g; Sodium: 204mg; Protein: 7g; Potassium: 145mg

HOMEMADE HASH BROWNS

SERVES 2 / PREP TIME: 5 MINUTES / COOK TIME: 25 MINUTES

Potato and chive crunchy hash browns.

---

1 MEDIUM WHITE POTATO, PEELED AND DICED

1 TBSP CHIVES

1 TBSP NON-FAT GREEK YOGURT

1 TSP UNSALTED BUTTER

---

1. Bring a pot of water to the boil over a high heat.
2. Add potato, lower heat slightly and allow to simmer for 10-15 minutes until soft.
3. Drain and remove from the pan.
4. Use a potato masher to mash potatoes in a mixing bowl and add chives and yogurt before mixing well.
5. Use your hands to shape the potato mixture into two patties.
6. Now melt the unsalted butter in a skillet over a medium heat.
7. Add each hash brown to the skillet and brown each side for 3-4 minutes.

Per serving: Calories: 94; Fat: 2g (Saturated Fat: 1g); Carbohydrates: 17g; Fiber: 2g; Sugar: 1g; Sodium: 206mg; Protein: 2g; Potassium: 289mg

PEACH CRÊPES

SERVES 2 / PREP TIME: 5 MINUTES / COOK TIME: 10 MINUTES

Sweet and scrumptious!

---

1 TBSP HONEY

1/4 CUP NON-FAT GREEK YOGURT

1 LARGE EGG YOLK

1/4 CUP WHITE FLOUR (GLUTEN-FREE IF NEEDED)

1/2 TSP BAKING POWDER

1 LARGE EGG WHITE

1 TSP UNSALTED BUTTER

1/4 CUP CANNED PEACHES, SKINLESS & UNSWEETENED

---

1. Heat the peaches in a skillet over a medium heat for 4-5 minutes to warm through.
2. Blend in a food processor to purée and place to one side.
3. Whisk the honey, Greek yogurt and egg yolk in a bowl.
4. Add the dry ingredients to a separate bowl and mix.
5. Gradually add the wet ingredients into the dry, whilst whisking until combined.
6. Now beat the egg white into soft peaks.
7. Fold the egg white into the batter.
8. Heat a skillet over a medium heat and melt the butter.
9. Pour 1/2 of the mixture in the skillet to form a pancake.
10. Cook for 2 minutes on each side or until cooked through and golden.
11. Repeat with the rest of the mixture.
12. Serve each crêpe with the puréed peach and a little sugar if desired.

Per serving: Calories: 226; Fat: 5g (Saturated Fat: 2g); Carbohydrates: 28g; Fiber: 1g; Sugar: 8g; Sodium: 267mg; Protein: 18g; Potassium: 278mg

CRANBERRY RICE PUDDING

SERVES 2 / PREP TIME: 5 MINUTES   COOK TIME: 10 MINUTES

So creamy and sweet!

1/2 CUP UNCOOKED WHITE RICE

1/4 CUP APPLE JUICE

1/2 CUP WATER

1/4 CUP RICE MILK

1 TBSP PURE HONEY

1 TSP GROUND NUTMEG

1 TSP VANILLA EXTRACT

1/4 CUP CANNED CRANBERRIES, SKIN-LESS& UNSWEETENED

---

1. Blend the rice in a food processor or grinder until powdered.
2. Add the juice, water, rice milk, honey, nutmeg and vanilla extract to a pan over a high heat and bring to the boil.
3. Gradually add the rice powder to the pan whilst stirring.
4. Turn down the heat and cover to simmer for 5 minutes.
5. Add the canned cranberries for 3 minutes or until hot through.
6. Stir before serving.

Per serving: Calories: 173; Fat: 1g (Saturated Fat: 0g); Carbohydrates: 40g; Fiber: 1g; Sugar: 27g; Sodium: 32mg; Protein: 1g; Potassium: 82mg

BREAKFAST BANANA MUFFINS

SERVES 2 / PREP TIME: 10 MINUTES / COOK TIME: 18 MINUTES

Delightful muffins to start your day!

---

2 TBSP NON-FAT SOUR CREAM

1/2 TSP VANILLA EXTRACT

1/2 TBSP CANOLA OIL

1 LARGE EGG WHITE

1/2 CUP WHITE FLOUR (GLUTEN-FREE IF NEEDED)

1/2 TSP BAKING POWDER

1 SMALL RIPE BANANA, PEELED AND SLICED

---

1. Preheat oven to 400°F/200 °C/Gas Mark 6.
2. Line a muffin tray with 4 muffin cases or lightly oil.
3. In a small bowl combine sour cream, vanilla extract, oil and egg white.
4. In a larger bowl, mix the dry ingredients together.
5. Now stir the wet ingredients into the dry ingredients.
6. Mix in the sliced banana.
7. Divide the batter into 4 muffin cases and then bake in the oven for 15-18 minutes or until cooked through.
8. Enjoy alone!

Hint: These muffins are great to pop in a lunch box for a breakfast on the go!

Per serving: Calories: 182; Fat:1g (Saturated Fat: 0g); Carbohydrates: 38g; Fiber: 2g; Sugar: 7g; Sodium: 198mg; Protein: 6g; Potassium: 263mg

RICE PUFF BIRCHER

SERVES 2 / PREP TIME: 5 MINUTES / COOK TIME: 30 MINUTES

Delicious smooth and crispy contrast!

1/2 CUP CANNED PEARS, SKINLESS & UNSWEETENED	**1 CUP WATER**
1 TSP NUTMEG	**1 CUP NON-FAT GREEK YOGURT**
1 TSP CINNAMON	**1/2 CUP RICE PUFF CEREAL (RICE KRISPIES TM)**
1 TSP STEVIA	

---

1. Add the pears, nutmeg, cinnamon, stevia and water to a pan over a high heat and bring to almost boiling point.
2. Reduce the heat, cover and simmer for 20-30 minutes or until reduced.
3. Remove from the pan and allow to cool.
4. Stir the rice puff cereal into the yogurt and then stir in the pear compote.
5. Cover and refrigerate overnight for a delicious bircher-style breakfast in the morning!

Hint: Alternatively serve the compote warm for a contrast in temperatures!

Per serving: Calories: 124; Fat: 1g (Saturated Fat: 0g); Carbohydrates: 18g; Fiber: 2g; Sugar: 10g; Sodium: 93mg; Protein: 14g; Potassium: 237mg

TURKEY SAUSAGE PATTIES

SERVES 2 / PREP TIME: 5 MINUTES / COOK TIME: 12 MINUTES

Scrumptious on a Sunday morning!

4OZ GROUND TURKEY

1/4 CUP CARROT, PEELED AND GRATED

1/2 TSP DRIED THYME

1 TBSP WATER

1 TSP OLIVE OIL

1/2 CUP MUSHROOMS, PEELED

---

1. Mix all of the ingredients in a large bowl (except the oil and mushrooms).
2. Wet your hands and shape the mixture into 2 flat patties.
3. Heat the oil in a skillet over a medium heat.
4. Cook the patties for 5-6 minutes on each side or until thoroughly cooked through.
5. Whilst cooking, add the mushrooms to the skillet and cook thoroughly.
6. Top the turkey patties with the mushrooms and enjoy!

Per serving: Calories: 60; Fat: 4g (Saturated Fat: 1g); Carbohydrates: 2g; Fiber: 1g; Sugar: 1g; Sodium: 25mg; Protein: 4g; Potassium: 138mg

CHEESE & PINEAPPLE BRUNCH

SERVES 2 / PREP TIME: 5 MINUTES / COOK TIME: 10 MINUTES

A fruity-cheesy accompaniment to your usual crackers!

1/2 CUP LOW FAT COTTAGE CHEESE

1/4 CUP CANNED PINEAPPLE (UN-SWEETENED), DICED

2 SALTINE CRACKERS

---

1. Sauté the pineapple in a skillet over a medium heat for 10 minutes.
2. Remove and allow to cool completely.
3. Mix together with the cottage cheese.
4. Serve with the crackers on the side for a healthy and filling brunch or snack.

Per serving: Calories: 71; Fat: 2g (Saturated Fat: 1g); Carbohydrates: 7g; Fiber: 0g; Sugar: 4g; Sodium: 215mg; Protein: 7g; Potassium: 91mg

SEAFOOD & POULTRY ENTRÉES

CHICKEN WITH CARROT & SQUASH PURÉE

SERVES 2 / PREP TIME: 5 MINUTES / COOK TIME: 30 MINUTES

Lightly spiced chicken with a sweet side.

1/4 CUP ACORN SQUASH PEELED AND CHOPPED

1 TSP GROUND NUTMEG

1/2 TSP BLACK PEPPER

1 SMALL CARROT, PEELED AND CHOPPED

1/2 TBSP OLIVE OIL

4OZ CHICKEN BREASTS, SKINLESS AND SLICED

1/2 TSP DRIED ROSEMARY

---

1. Bring a pot of water to the boil and add the squash, nutmeg and black pepper.
2. Cook for 25-30 minutes or until very soft.
3. Add the carrots for the last 20 minutes.
4. Meanwhile, heat the oil in a skillet over a medium-high heat.
5. Add the sliced chicken and stir to brown.
6. Sprinkle over the rosemary and continue to sauté for 20 minutes.
7. Check chicken is thoroughly cooked through - it should not be pink in the middle.
8. Drain vegetables and allow to cool slightly.
9. Blend in a food processor until smooth.
10. Serve sliced chicken on a helping of purée and enjoy.

Per serving: Calories: 74; Fat: 4g (Saturated Fat: 1); Carbohydrates: 4g; Fiber: 1g; Sugar: 1g; Sodium: 83mg; Protein: 5g; Potassium: 173mg

MOUTH-WATERING MEATBALLS

SERVES 2 / PREP TIME: 5 MINUTES / COOK TIME: 30 MINUTES

A wholesome and fulfilling meatball dish that the whole family will enjoy!

4OZ LEAN GROUND TURKEY

1 TBSP FRESH PARSLEY, CHOPPED

1 LARGE EGG WHITE

1 TSP OLIVE OIL

1 TBSP LOW SODIUM TOMATO PASTE

1/4 CUP WATER

1/2 CUP MUSHROOMS, SLICED

---

1. Mix the ground turkey with the parsley and egg white.
2. Use the palms of your hands to form 8 meatballs.
3. Heat the oil in a skillet over a medium-high heat and add the meatballs.
4. Brown by carefully turning with a cooking spoon for 5-10 minutes.
5. Now mix the tomato paste and water together until combined.
6. Pour over the meatballs and bring to a simmer.
7. Add the mushrooms into the sauce and allow to simmer on a low heat for 10 minutes.
8. Check meatballs are cooked through by slicing into one and ensuring there is no pink meat.
9. Serve the meatballs and sauce piping hot!

Hint: The meatballs can be made in bulk in the sauce and frozen for 2-3 weeks. Simply portion up and then pull a portion from the freezer and allow to thoroughly defrost before heating though in a pan when ready to cook!

Per serving: Calories: 155; Fat: 9g (Saturated Fat: 2g); Carbohydrates: 2g; Fiber: 1g; Sugar: 1g; Sodium: 111mg; Protein: 17g; Potassium: 314mg

HERBY CHICKEN & SQUASH STEW

SERVES 2 / PREP TIME: 10 MINUTES / COOK TIME: 40 MINUTES

A tasty Mediterranean inspired dish.

---

1 TSP OLIVE OIL

1/4 CUP ACORN SQUASH, PEELED AND CUBED

1 SMALL CARROT, PEELED AND DICED

1/2 CUP LOW SODIUM CHICKEN STOCK

1 CUP WATER

1/2 TSP DRIED THYME

1/2 TSP DRIED TARRAGON

1 BAY LEAF

4OZ CHICKEN BREAST, BONELESS & SKINLESS

---

1. Preheat a medium sized Dutch oven or large pot over a medium heat on the stove.
2. Add olive oil, squash cubes and carrots.
3. Stir and cook 3 minutes.
4. Now stir in the stock, water, herbs and bay leaf.
5. Bring to a boil, cover and simmer for 15 minutes or until vegetables are tender.
6. Add the chicken cubes and return to a simmer until cooked through (approximately 15-20 minutes).
7. Serve hot right away or allow to cool slightly and blend into a smooth soup.
8. Season with pepper to taste.

Per serving: Calories: 135 Fat: 5g (Saturated Fat: 1g); Carbohydrates: 5g; Fiber: 1g; Sugar: 1g; Sodium: 308mg; Protein: 18g; Potassium: 379mg

POLLOCK EN PAPILLOTE

SERVES 2 / PREP TIME: 5 MINUTES / COOK TIME: 25 MINUTES

Flaky white fish with potatoes - a taste of home!

---

1 SMALL WHITE POTATO, PEELED AND CUBED

1 SHEET PARCHMENT PAPER

4OZ POLLOCK FILLET, SKINLESS AND DE-BONED (OR OTHER WHITE FISH OF CHOICE)

1 TSP OLIVE OIL

1 TBSP FRESH PARSLEY

---

1. Preheat the oven to 190°C/375°F/Gas Mark 5.
2. Bring a small pot of water to the boil over a high heat.
3. Add the cubed potato and lower the heat slightly.
4. Cook for 15-20 minutes or until very soft.
5. Meanwhile, lay out the parchment paper on an oven tray.
6. Place the pollock fillet onto the paper and drizzle over the olive oil.
7. Add the parsley.
8. Fold the paper over and lightly scrunch the edges together to make a loose parcel.
9. Add to the oven for 15-18 minutes or until fish is thoroughly cooked through and flakes easily.
10. Now drain the potato, season to taste and serve on the side of half of the fish.
11. Enjoy!

Per serving: Calories: 119; Fat: 3g (Saturated Fat: 0g); Carbohydrates: 13g; Fiber: 1g; Sugar: 1g; Sodium: 186mg; Protein: 11g; Potassium: 319mg

FRAGRANT CHICKEN CURRY

SERVES 2 / PREP TIME: 5 MINUTES / COOK TIME: 30 MINUTES

A mild yet fragrant chicken curry.

4OZ CHICKEN BREAST, BONELESS &
SKINLESS

1/2 TBSP GARLIC INFUSED OIL

1 TSP SWEET CURRY POWDER

1 TBSP TOMATO PASTE

1 BAY LEAF

1 CINNAMON STICK

1/2 CUP LOW SODIUM CHICKEN STOCK

1 CUP WATER

1 TBSP FRESH CILANTRO, CHOPPED

---

1. Dice the chicken into bite-size cubes.
2. Heat a large wok or pot over a medium heat.
3. Add the oil to melt.
4. Sauté chicken pieces until golden brown.
5. Now add the curry powder, tomato paste, bay leaf, cinnamon stick, water and chicken stock.
6. Simmer for 20 minutes.
7. Ensure the chicken is thoroughly cooked through before serving with the fresh cilantro scattered over the top.
8. Enjoy with white rice or bread to mop up the flavors.

Per serving: Calories: 139; Fat: 6g (Saturated Fat: 1g); Carbohydrates: 3g; Fiber: 1g; Sugar: 1g; Sodium: 299mg; Protein: 19g; Potassium: 356mg

CREAMY CHICKEN & MUSHROOM SOUP

SERVES 2 / PREP TIME: 5 MINUTES / COOK TIME: 15 MINUTES

A winter warmer.

4OZ ROASTED AND SKINLESS CHICKEN BREAST

1/2 CUP LOW-SODIUM CHICKEN STOCK

1 CUP WATER

1/4 CUP COOKED EGG NOODLES

1 CUP MUSHROOMS, COOKED

1 TSP DRIED DILL

1 TSP DRIED THYME

1 TSP BLACK PEPPER

1/4 CUP SKIM MILK (OR DAIRY-FREE EQUIVALENT)

---

1. Use leftover chicken or alternatively, roast the chicken in foil in the oven for 25-30 minutes or until thoroughly cooked through prior to preparing the soup. (Heat oven to 190°C/375°F/Gas Mark 5 to cook).
2. Slice the chicken.
3. Now add the stock and water to a pot over a high heat and bring to the boil.
4. Add the chicken, noodles, mushrooms, herbs and pepper.
5. Turn down the heat slightly, stir in the milk, and allow to simmer for 10 minutes.
6. Remove from the heat and allow to cool slightly.
7. Blend in food processor for a smooth, creamy soup.

Hint: No need to blend if you can handle solid foods.

Per serving: Calories: 133; Fat: 5.5g (Saturated Fat: 0g); Carbohydrates: 13g; Fiber: 2g; Sugar: 3g; Sodium: 133.5mg; Protein: 21.5g

PARSLEY BUTTER HADDOCK

SERVES 2 / PREP TIME: 5 MINUTES / COOK TIME: 30 MINUTES

Buttery poached fish with crushed petite potatoes.

1/2 CUP PEELED PETITE POTATOES

4OZ HADDOCK FILLET, DE-BONED AND SKINLESS (OR OTHER WHITE FISH)

2 CUPS SKIM MILK (OR DAIRY-FREE)

1 TBSP UNSALTED BUTTER (USE OLIVE OIL IF LACTOSE INTOLERANT)

1/4 CUP FRESH PARSLEY, CHOPPED

---

1. Bring a pot of water to the boil and add the peeled baby potatoes.
2. Lower the heat slightly and allow to simmer for 15-20 minutes.
3. Meanwhile, add the milk to a separate pot over a medium-high heat.
4. Add the haddock and allow to poach in the milk for 15-20 minutes or until thoroughly cooked through.
5. Drain potatoes and haddock (reserve 1 tbsp of the milk).
6. Use a fork to crush the potatoes with the reserved milk.
7. Heat the butter in a skillet over a medium heat.
8. Add the chopped parsley to the skillet once melted.
9. Plate up the potatoes and haddock and drizzle over the delicious parsley butter.
10. Season with pepper to taste.
11. Enjoy!

Per serving: Calories: 150; Fat: 6g (Saturated Fat: 4g); Carbohydrates: 12g; Fiber: 1g; Sugar: 1g; Sodium: 179mg; Protein: 11g; Potassium: 345mg

SCALLOPS & APPLE

SERVES 2 / PREP TIME: 5 MINUTES / COOK TIME: 5 MINUTES

Simple yet so sweet!

5OZ FRESH KING SCALLOPS

1 TBSP UNSALTED BUTTER/OLIVE OIL

1 TSP CURRY POWDER

2 TBSP APPLE SAUCE

---

1. Melt the butter/oil in a skillet over a medium heat.
2. Add the scallops, browning each side for 1-2 minutes.
3. Heat the apple sauce in the microwave or a separate skillet.
4. Sprinkle scallops with curry powder and serve with the apple sauce.
5. Enjoy as a starter or lunch time treat.

Per serving: Calories: 155; Fat: 7g (Saturated Fat: 4g); Carbohydrates: 9g; Fiber: 1g; Sugar: 5g; Sodium: 370mg; Protein: 15g; Potassium: 327mg

SAGE & SPINACH STUFFED TURKEY BREASTS

SERVES 2 / PREP TIME: 5 MINUTES / COOK TIME: 35 MINUTES

A Thanksgiving or Christmas staple but feel free to enjoy any time of the year!

4OZ TURKEY BREAST, SKINLESS & SLICED IN HALF)

2 SHEETS OF PLASTIC WRAP

1 TSP UNSALTED BUTTER/OLIVE OIL

1 TSP GROUND NUTMEG

1 CUP FROZEN SPINACH

1 TSP DRIED SAGE

1 SALTINE CRACKER, CRUSHED

---

1. Preheat oven to 375°F/190 °C/Gas Mark 5.
2. Butterfly each turkey breast piece and place flat on the left edge of a sheet of plastic wrap.
3. Fold the right edge of the plastic wrap over the turkey and use a rolling pin or meat pounder to flatten to 1/2 cm thick.
4. Repeat for the second piece.
5. Heat the butter/oil in a skillet over a medium heat and add the spinach and nutmeg for 5-10 minutes or until the spinach is thoroughly cooked.
6. Remove from the heat and mix with the crushed crackers and sage in a separate bowl.
7. Unfold the plastic wrap and spread the stuffing over the turkey breasts.
8. Now pick up the corners of the plastic wrap closest to you and carefully roll the turkey away from you.
9. Add the turkey rolls to an oven dish filled with hot water.
10. Place in the oven for 25-30 minutes or until thoroughly cooked through.
11. Serve hot with your choice of side.

Per serving: Calories: 94; Fat: 3g (Saturated Fat: 2g); Carbohydrates: 3g; Fiber: 2g; Sugar: 1g; Sodium:70mg; Protein: 14g; Potassium: 275mg

SHRIMP SPAGHETTI

SERVES 2 / PREP TIME: 5 MINUTES / COOK TIME: 20 MINUTES

A taste of the Mediterranean!

1/2 CUP (4OZ) SPAGHETTI NOODLES

1 TSP OLIVE OIL

4OZ SHRIMP

1 TBSP LOW SODIUM TOMATO PASTE

1/4 CUP HOMEMADE FISH/VEGETABLE STOCK

1 TBSP FRESH CILANTRO, CHOPPED

---

1. Bring a pot of water to the boil over a high heat.
2. Add the pasta, lower the heat, and allow to simmer for 10-15 minutes or according to package directions.
3. In a separate skillet, add the olive oil and sauté the shrimp over a medium heat for 10 minutes or until shrimp turns opaque.
4. Stir in the tomato paste and stock and allow to simmer for a further 10 minutes.
5. Drain the pasta and add to the skillet with the shrimps.
6. Toss to mix.
7. Sprinkle with cilantro to serve.

Per serving: Calories: 287; Fat: 4g (Saturated Fat: 1g); Carbohydrates: 43g; Fiber: 3g; Sugar: 2g; Sodium: 565mg; Protein: 18g; Potassium: 207mg

GINGERED CLAM NOODLES

SERVES 2 / PREP TIME: 5 MINUTES / COOK TIME: 25 MINUTES

A hint of the orient.

1/2 CUP EGG NOODLES	4OZ CLAMS
1 TSP COCONUT OIL	1 TSP GINGER PASTE
1/2 CUP MUSHROOMS	1 TBSP CHINESE FLAT LEAF PARSLEY

1. Cook the egg noodles in a pan of boiling water (1 cup) for 10-15 minutes or according to package directions.
2. Meanwhile, heat the oil in a skillet over a medium-high heat and add the mushrooms.
3. Sauté for 10 minutes until thoroughly cooked through.
4. Now add the clams, cook for 5-10 minutes or until cooked through.
5. Now add the ginger paste and stir.
6. Drain the noodles and top with the shrimp and mushrooms.
7. Sprinkle over the Chinese flat-leaf parsley and serve.

Per serving: Calories: 116; Fat: 4g (Saturated Fat: 2g); Carbohydrates: 16g; Fiber: 1g; Sugar: 1g; Sodium: 90mg; Protein: 5g; Potassium: 155mg

PEANUT TURKEY SATAY

SERVES 2 / PREP TIME: 10 MINUTES / COOK TIME: 35 MINUTES

Nutty and delicious!

---

1 TBSP SMOOTH PEANUT BUTTER

1 TBSP WATER

1 TBSP LOW SODIUM TOMATO PASTE

4OZ TURKEY BREAST, SKINLESS

1/2 CUP WHITE RICE

1 TBSP FRESH CILANTRO, CHOPPED

---

1. Mix the peanut butter with the water and tomato paste to make a satay sauce.
2. Cut the turkey into cubes and marinate in the satay sauce for as long as possible.
3. Preheat the broiler to a medium-high heat.
4. Add the turkey to a lined baking tray, and drizzle over the marinade.
5. Place under the broiler for 25-30 minutes or until turkey is thoroughly cooked through.
6. Meanwhile, add the rice to a pan of cold water (1 cup) and bring to the boil over a high heat.
7. Lower the heat and simmer for 20 minutes or until most of the water is absorbed.
8. Drain and cover to steam for 5 minutes.
9. Serve the satay turkey on a bed of white rice and sprinkle with cilantro to serve.

Per serving: Calories: 282; Fat: 5g (Saturated Fat: 1g); Carbohydrates: 41g; Fiber: 1g; Sugar: 2g; Sodium: 55mg; Protein: 18g; Potassium: 307mg

SEA BASS WITH BASIL MASH POTATO

SERVES 2 / PREP TIME: 10 MINUTES / COOK TIME: 30 MINUTES

What a treat!

---

1 WHITE POTATO, PEELED AND DICED

1 TBSP OLIVE OIL

1/4 CUP FRESH BASIL, FINELY CHOPPED

1 TBSP UNSALTED BUTTER

4OZ SEA BASS FILLET, SKINLESS

---

1. Place the potato and 1 tbsp olive oil in a microwavable zip lock bag.
2. Place this into the microwave for 20 minutes (alternatively, boil in a pot for 25 minutes).
3. Meanwhile, heat 1 tbsp olive oil in a skillet over a medium-high heat and cook the sea bass fillet for 6 minutes.
4. Turn and cook the over side for 4 minutes (ensure fish is thoroughly cooked through).
5. Remove from the heat and place to one side.
6. Once cooked, remove the potato from the microwave and very carefully unzip the bag (it will be steaming hot).
7. Pop the potato into a large bowl and mash with a potato masher.
8. Mix in the chopped basil and butter and allow to melt.
9. Gently flake the sea bass fillet and serve on top of the basil mash.

Hint: Use olive oil instead of butter if lactose intolerant.

Per serving: Calories: 228; Fat: 13g (Saturated Fat: 5g); Carbohydrates: 17g; Fiber: 2g; Sugar: 1g; Sodium: 237mg; Protein: 11g; Potassium: 395mg

VEGETARIAN ENTRÉES

TOFU SCRAMBLE

SERVES 2 / PREP TIME: 5 MINUTES / COOK TIME: 20 MINUTES

Delicious vegetarian meal.

1 TSP COCONUT OIL

1 CUP SILKEN TOFU, CUBED

1 TSP GINGER PASTE

1/4 CUP MUSHROOMS

1/4 CUP SPINACH

1. Heat the coconut oil in a wok or non-stick skillet over a high heat.
2. Add the tofu and ginger paste and brown for 5-10 minutes.
3. Add the mushrooms and spinach for 10 minutes or until thoroughly cooked through.
4. Serve hot with your choice of rice or noodles.

Per serving: Calories: 101; Fat: 7g (Saturated Fat: 3g); Carbohydrates: 3g; Fiber: 1g; Sugar: 1g; Sodium: 14mg; Protein: 9g; Potassium; 209mg

VEGETARIAN MINI LASAGNA

SERVES 2 / PREP TIME: 10 MINUTES / COOK TIME: 30 MINUTES

A tasty baked vegetarian pasta dish.

1/4 CUP ACORN SQUASH, SLICED

1 CUP SPINACH

FOR THE WHITE SAUCE:

1 TBSP UNSALTED BUTTER

1 OZ CUP WHITE FLOUR (GF IF NEEDED)

1 CUP SKIM MILK OR EQUIVALENT

---

1. Preheat the oven to 350°f/170°c/Gas Mark 4.
2. Make the white sauce: heat the butter in a small pan over a low-medium heat.
3. Tilt the pan towards you so that the butter melts only on the near side of the pan as much as possible.
4. Add the flour to the far side of the pan and slowly mix this into the melted butter using a wooden spoon.
5. Once a paste is formed, add the milk slowly and stir continuously for approximately 10-15 minutes or until the lumps disappear (don't worry, they will!)
6. Now, line a small/medium sized lasagna dish with 1/3 squash slices.
7. Create the next layer with 1/3 spinach.
8. Top with 1/3 white sauce.
9. Repeat 2 more layers with the rest of the ingredients and place in the oven for 30 minutes or until golden and bubbling.
10. Enjoy!

Per serving: Calories: 155; Fat: 6g (Saturated Fat: 4g); Carbohydrates: 19g; Fiber: 1g; Sugar: 6g; Sodium: 65mg; Protein: 6g Potassium; 352mg

SPINACH HASH CAKES

SERVES 2 / PREP TIME: 5 MINUTES / COOK TIME: 30 MINUTES

Golden and crispy potato treats.

---

1 CUP SPINACH

1 MEDIUM WHITE POTATO, PEELED AND CUBED

1 TBSP UNSALTED BUTTER/OLIVE OIL

---

1. Place all ingredients into a microwavable zip lock bag.
2. Place this into the microwave for 20 minutes. Alternatively, boil in a pot for 25 minutes.
3. Remove the potato from the microwave and very carefully unzip the bag (it will be steaming hot).
4. Pop the potato and spinach mixture into a large bowl and mash with a potato masher.
5. Use wet hands to form palm size 'cakes'.
6. Heat the broiler on high.
7. Add the cakes to a baking tray and cook for 4 minutes on each side or until golden and slightly crispy.
8. Enjoy!

Per serving: Calories: 125; Fat: 6g (Saturated Fat: 4g); Carbohydrates: 17g; Fiber: 2g; Sugar: 1g; Sodium: 215g; Protein: 2g; Potassium; 358mg

BAKED BEETS & RICOTTA FRITTATA

SERVES 2 / PREP TIME: 5 MINUTES / COOK TIME: 10 MINUTES

A vibrant treat.

1/2 CUP CANNED BEETS, SLICED

4 LARGE EGG WHITES

1/4 CUP SKIM MILK

1/4 CUP SKIM RICOTTA

1 TSP DRIED THYME

---

1. Turn the broiler on high.
2. Layer a tart dish or oven-proof skillet with the sliced beets.
3. Whisk up the egg whites and milk and pour over the beets.
4. Spoon the ricotta evenly over the top - don't worry if it sinks.
5. Place under the broiler for 10 minutes or until the eggs are cooked through and form an omelet consistency.
6. Remove, slice, sprinkle with thyme and enjoy!

Per serving: Calories: 99; Fat: 3g (Saturated Fat: 2g); Carbohydrates: 7g; Fiber: 1g; Sugar: 4g; Sodium: 345mg; Protein: 12g; Potassium; 260mg

ACORN SQUASH RISOTTO

SERVES 2 / PREP TIME: 5 MINUTES / COOK TIME: 30 MINUTES

Scrumptious and filling.

1/4 CUP ACORN SQUASH, PEELED AND CUBED

1 CUP VEGETABLE STOCK

1 CUP WATER

2 SPRIGS THYME

1 TBSP OLIVE OIL

1/2 CUP MUSHROOMS, SLICED

1/2 CUP WHITE RICE

2 TBSP FAT FREE GREEK YOGURT

---

1. Add the cubed squash to a pan of water and bring to the boil.
2. Allow to boil for 20-25 minutes or until soft.
3. Meanwhile, add the stock, water, thyme and rice to a separate pot and simmer over a medium heat until the liquid has been absorbed (25 minutes). Then drain.
4. Once the squash is cooked, heat the oil in a large pan or wok over a medium-high heat.
5. Now add the mushrooms and stir.
6. Mix in the rice and squash.
7. Top with the Greek yogurt to serve.

Per serving: Calories: 259; Fat: 7g (Saturated Fat: 1g); Carbohydrates: 42g; Fiber: 1g; Sugar: 1g; Sodium: 397mg; Protein: 6g;Potassium; 208mg

EGG RAMEN NOODLES

SERVES 2 / PREP TIME: 5 MINUTES / COOK TIME: 20 MINUTES

A vegetarian take on a traditional Eastern dish.

1/4 CUP MUSHROOMS

1/4 CUP SPINACH

1 LARGE HARD BOILED EGG

1/2 CUP LOW SODIUM VEGETABLE STOCK

1 CUP COOKED EGG NOODLES

1 TSP CHINESE FIVE- SPICE

1 TBSP PARSLEY, FRESHLY CHOPPED

---

1. Cook mushrooms and spinach in a skillet for 10 minutes or until well cooked. Add a little oil if necessary to prevent sticking.
2. Meanwhile, boil the egg in a pot of boiling water for 5-6 minutes.
3. Rinse under the cold tap and remove the shell carefully.
4. Place veg and egg to one side.
5. In a pot, bring the stock to a simmer over a medium heat.
6. Add the noodles, spinach and mushrooms and lower the heat slightly.
7. Sprinkle in the Chinese five-spice.
8. Allow to simmer for 5-10 minutes.
9. Once piping hot, remove and serve with half a boiled egg each and a sprinkle of parsley.

Per serving: Calories: 119; Fat: 4g (Saturated Fat: 1g); Carbohydrates: 15g; Fiber: 1g; Sugar: 1g; Sodium: 224mg; Protein: 7g; Potassium; 128mg

VEGETABLE CHINESE-SPICED STIR FRY

SERVES 2 / PREP TIME: 5 MINUTES / COOK TIME: 20 MINUTES

A light and fulfilling noodle dish.

---

1 MEDIUM CARROT, PEELED

1 SMALL ZUCCHINI, PEELED

1 CUP EGG NOODLES

1 TSP CANOLA OIL

1 TSP RAW HONEY

1 TSP CHINESE FIVE-SPICE

---

1. Cut the carrot and zucchini into thin strips or batons.
2. Cook the noodles according to package directions.
3. Heat the oil in a skillet over a medium-high heat.
4. Add the carrots, zucchini, honey and five-spice.
5. Stir fry for 10 minutes.
6. Drain the noodles and add to the pan with the rest of the ingredients.
7. Serve hot and enjoy.

Per serving: Calories: 129; Fat: 4g (Saturated Fat: 0g); Carbohydrates: 21g; Fiber: 2g; Sugar: 6g; Sodium: 29mg; Protein: 4g; Potassium; 274mg

RAINBOW RICE SALAD

SERVES 2 / PREP TIME: 5 MINUTES / COOK TIME: 20 MINUTES

Try serving hot or cold!

1/2 CUP WHITE RICE

1 TSP OLIVE OIL

1/4 CUP ZUCCHINI, PEELED & SLICED

2 OZ SILKEN TOFU, CUBED

1/4 CUP CANNED BEETS, SLICED

1 TSP DRIED BASIL

1 TSP DRIED DILL

---

1. Cook the rice according to package directions.
2. Meanwhile, heat the oil in a skillet over a medium-high heat.
3. Add the rest of the ingredients (minus the herbs) and sauté for 10-15 minutes or until thoroughly cooked through.
4. Mix the vegetables through the rice and serve with the fresh herbs.

Per serving: Calories: 223; Fat: 4g (Saturated Fat: 1g); Carbohydrates: 41g; Fiber: 1g; Sugar: 2g; Sodium: 48mg; Protein: 6g; Potassium; 184mg

ZUCCHINI MINT & CHIVE SOUP

SERVES 2 / PREP TIME: 5 MINUTES / COOK TIME: 20 MINUTES

Light and refreshing!

1/2 CUP LOW-SODIUM VEGETABLE STOCK

1 CUP WATER

1 CUP ZUCCHINI, PEELED AND DICED

1 TBSP MINT, FRESHLY CHOPPED

1 TBSP FRESH CHIVES, CHOPPED

---

1. Add the stock and water to a large pot over a medium heat and bring to a simmer.
2. Add the zucchini for 5-10 minutes or until thoroughly cooked through.
3. Now add the mint and cook for a further 5 minutes.
4. Allow to cool slightly and blend in a food processor until smooth.
5. Sprinkle in the chives and enjoy hot!

Per serving: Calories: 23; Fat: 0g (Saturated Fat: 0); Carbohydrates: 4g; Fiber: 1g; Sugar: 3g; Sodium: 187mg; Protein: 1g; Potassium; 192mg

CARROT SOUP

SERVES 2 / PREP TIME: 10 MINUTES / COOK TIME: 35 MINUTES

A traditional soup.

1/2 CUP LOW-SODIUM VEGETABLE STOCK

1 CUP WATER

1 CUP CARROTS, PEELED AND CHOPPED

1 TSP GINGER PASTE

1 TSP FRESH CILANTRO

---

1. Bring the stock and water to a simmer and add the carrots along with the ginger paste.
2. Simmer for 30-35 minutes or until carrots are very soft.
3. Keep an eye on the soup and top up with water if it starts to dry out.
4. Allow to cool, then blend in a food processor until smooth.
5. Serve with fresh cilantro, season to taste, and enjoy.

Per serving: Calories: 35; Fat: 0g (Saturated Fat: 0g); Carbohydrates: 7g; Fiber: 2g; Sugar: 3g; Sodium: 231mg; Protein: 1g; Potassium; 208mg

MUSHROOM & TARRAGON SOUP

SERVES 2 / PREP TIME: 5 MINUTES / COOK TIME: 30 MINUTES

Light and tasty!

---

1 TBSP UNSALTED BUTTER/OLIVE OIL

1 TBSP TARRAGON FRESH OR DRIED

1 CUP RAW BUTTON MUSHROOMS, CHOPPED

1 TBSP PLAIN WHITE FLOUR (GF IF NEEDED)

1/2 CUP LOW SODIUM VEGETABLE STOCK

1 CUP SKIM MILK

---

1. Melt the butter/oil in a large pot over a medium heat.
2. Turn the heat up slightly and add the mushrooms for 5 minutes.
3. Add the tarragon and stir well.
4. Sprinkle the flour over the mushrooms and stir for 2 minutes.
5. Add the stock to the pot and simmer for 5 minutes.
6. Now add the milk slowly until combined.
7. Bring to the boil, turn down the heat and allow to simmer for 20 minutes.
8. Allow to cool slightly before blending in a food processor until smooth.
9. Serve!

Per serving: Calories: 121; Fat: 6g (Saturated Fat: 4g); Carbohydrates: 11g; Fiber: 1g; Sugar: 7g; Sodium: 241mg; Protein:6g; Potassium; 349mg

STOCKS & SAUCES

LOW SODIUM CHICKEN STOCK

SERVES: 16 CUPS / PREP TIME: 5 MINUTES / COOK TIME: 3-4 HOURS

Try this instead of shop bought stock!

BONES OF 1 WHOLE CHICKEN

1/2 CUP CARROTS, PEELED AND CHOPPED

2 TBSP THYME

1 TSP SEA SALT

8 CUPS WATER

1 BAY LEAF

1 ZUCCHINI, PEELED AND CHOPPED

---

1. Add all ingredients to a large pot on a medium heat and simmer for 3-4 hours.
2. Alternatively add to a slow cooker and cook on low for 12 hours.
3. Strain the stock through a fine sieve.
4. Allow to cool and then add to a sealed container in the refrigerator.
5. Use a spoon or knife to skim away any fat from the top before using or heat through thoroughly for a lovely broth to sip on.
6. You can freeze this in portions for up to 2-3 weeks and allow to defrost before use.

Hint: As homemade stock is high in calories and good fats but low in fiber, it can be sipped on throughout the day. Just don't forget to include in your daily calculations!

Please note: Each serving should be no more than 1/2 cup. If using in dishes, allocate 1/2 cup stock per person and use water to combine.

Per serving (1/2 cup) approx: Calories: 126; Fat: 7g (Saturated Fat: 2g); Carbohydrates: 1.25g; Fiber: 0g; Sugar: 0.5g; Sodium: 50.5mg; Protein: 13.5g

LOW SODIUM VEGETABLE STOCK

SERVES 8 CUPS / PREP TIME: 5 MINUTES / COOK TIME: 3-4 HOURS

Try using for homemade soups or stews.

---

1 CUP CARROTS, PEELED AND SLICED

1 CELERY STALK, CHOPPED

1 CUP MUSHROOMS, SLICED

8 CUPS WATER

1 TSP SEA SALT

1 TSP PARSLEY

2 TSP ROSEMARY, CHOPPED

1 BAY LEAF

1 TSP CUMIN

---

1. Add all ingredients to a large pot on a medium heat and simmer for 3-4 hours.
2. Alternatively add to a slow cooker and cook on low for 12 hours.
3. Strain the stock through a fine sieve.
4. Allow to cool and then add to a sealed container in the refrigerator.
5. Use a spoon or knife to skim away any fat from the top before using or heat through thoroughly for a lovely broth to sip on.
6. You can freeze this in portions for up to 2-3 weeks and allow to defrost before use.

Hint: As homemade stock is high in calories and good fats but low in fiber, it can be sipped on throughout the day. Just don't forget to include in your daily calculations!

Please note: Each serving should be no more than 1/2 cup. If using in dishes, allocate 1/2 cup stock per person and use water to combine.

Per serving (1/2 cup) approx: Calories: 9; Fat: 0g (Saturated Fat: 0g); Carbohydrates: 1.5g; Fiber: 0.5g; Sugar: 1g; Sodium: 50mg; Protein: 0g

LOW SODIUM FISH STOCK

SERVES 10 CUPS / PREP TIME: 15 MINUTES / COOK TIME: 3-4 HOURS

This tastes amazing in curries or added to noodles.

---

8 CUPS SHELLFISH (TRIMMINGS ARE FINE - ASK AT YOUR LOCAL FISHMONGER OR SUPERMARKET)

1 TSP SEA SALT

10 CUPS WATER

1 CELERY STALK, CHOPPED

1 TSP PARSLEY

1 TSP CILANTRO

3 CARROTS, PEELED AND CHOPPED

---

1. Add all of the ingredients to a large pot over a medium heat.
2. Simmer for 3-4 hours. Alternatively use a slow cooker to free you from the kitchen and simmer on low overnight).
3. Strain the broth through a sieve.
4. Allow to cool and store in a sealable container in the fridge for 2-3 days or in the freezer for 2-3 weeks.

Please note: Each serving should be no more than 1/2 cup. If using in dishes, allocate 1/2 cup stock per person and use water to combine.

Per serving (1/2 cup) approx: Calories: 34.5; Fat: 0.5g (Saturated Fat: 0g); Carbohydrates: 3.5g; Fiber: 0.5g; Sugar: 1.5; Sodium: 45mg; Protein: 0.5g

BONE BROTH

SERVES 8 CUPS / PREP TIME: 5 MINUTES / COOK TIME: 3-4 HOURS

Simply sip from a mug throughout the day.

---

5 BEEF BONES	1 TSP CINNAMON
1 CUP CARROTS, CHOPPED	1 CELERY STALK, CHOPPED
1 TSP SEA SALT	10 CUPS WATER
1 BAY LEAF	
1 TSP NUTMEG	

---

1. Add all ingredients to a large pot on a medium heat and simmer for 3-4 hours.
2. Alternatively add to a slow cooker and cook on low for 12 hours.
3. Strain the broth through a fine sieve.
4. Allow to cool and then add to a sealed container in the refrigerator.
5. Use a spoon or knife to skim away any fat that has stored as a layer on the top.
6. You can freeze this in portions for up to 2-3 weeks and allow to defrost before use.

Please note: Each serving should be no more than 1/2 cup. If using in dishes, allocate 1/2 cup stock per person and use water to combine.

Per serving (1/2 cup) approx: Calories: 34.5; Fat: 2g (Saturated Fat: 1g); Carbohydrates: 0.5g; Fiber: 0g; Sugar: 0g; Sodium: 45mg; Protein: 3g

HOMEMADE TOMATO SAUCE

SERVES 10 / PREP TIME: 10 MINUTES / COOK TIME: 15 MINUTES

A great dipping sauce or add to pasta dishes.

---

5 CUPS LARGE VERY RIPE TOMATOES

1 TSP OREGANO

1 TSP BASIL

---

1. Cover the tomatoes with boiling water in a large bowl.
2. Leave for 3 minutes and drain.
3. Rinse with cold water before peeling skins off.
4. Quarter and de-seed tomatoes with a knife and then press the rest through a strainer or sieve to get rid of any pulp.
5. Do the same with the seeds from earlier to get as much juice as you can from them!
6. Add to a small pan on a medium heat and sprinkle with the herbs.
7. Allow to simmer for 10-15 minutes or until hot through.
8. Alternatively serve cold!

Per serving: Calories:33; Fat: 0g (Saturated Fat: 0g); Carbohydrates: 8g; Fiber: 1g; Sugar: 4g; Sodium: 282mg; Protein: 1g; Potassium: 264

HOMEMADE BECHAMEL SAUCE

SERVES 5 / PREP TIME: 15 MINUTES / COOK TIME: 10 MINUTES

Try with lasagna or fish.

1 TBSP UNSALTED BUTTER

1 OZ WHITE FLOUR (GF IF NEEDED)

1 CUP SKIM MILK OR EQUIVALENT

1. Heat the butter in a small pan over a low-medium heat.
2. Tilt the pan towards you so that the butter melts only on the near side of the pan as much as possible.
3. Add the flour to the far side of the pan and slowly mix this into the melted butter using a wooden spoon.
4. Once a paste is formed, add the milk slowly and stir continuously for approximately 5 minutes or until the lumps disappear (don't worry, they will!)

Per serving: Calories: 58; Fat: 2g (Saturated Fat: 1g); Carbohydrates: 7g; Fiber: 0g; Sugar: 3g; Sodium: 21mg; Protein: 2g; Potassium: 83

GINGER PASTE

SERVES 10 / PREP TIME: 5 MINUTES / COOK TIME: N/A

Add to your stir-fries, poultry or even yogurts for a bit of a kick!

---

2 WHOLE GINGER ROOTS, PEELED AND SLICED

1 CUP WATER

---

1. Add the ginger and water to a food processor until smooth.
2. Strain through a sieve to get rid of any fibrous strands.
3. Repeat if necessary.
4. Keep in a sealed container in the fridge for 2-3 days or add to an ice cube tray and simple pop into your dishes to add a little kick!

Per serving: Calories: 4; Fat: 0g (Saturated Fat: 0g); Carbohydrates: 0g; Fiber: 0g; Sugar: 0g; Sodium: 0mg; Protein: 0g

HOMEMADE GRAVY

SERVES 10 / PREP TIME: 5 MINUTES / COOK TIME: 20 MINUTES

A low sodium alternative to shop bought gravy.

---

1 TBSP OLIVE OIL

1 CUP CARROTS, PEELED, CHOPPED AND BOILED

2 CUPS LOW SODIUM CHICKEN STOCK

2 CUPS WATER

1 TSP FRESH OR DRIED TARRAGON

1 TBSP FRESH OR DRIED PARSLEY

---

1. Add the oil to a large pot over a medium heat.
2. Add the carrots for 1-2 minutes.
3. Add the rest of the ingredients and allow to simmer for 20 minutes or until thickened.
4. Serve right away or allow to cool before adding to a sealed container and storing in the fridge for 2-3 days.
5. Alternatively you can freeze the gravy and defrost when you need it!

Per serving: Calories: 25; Fat:2g (Saturated Fat: 0g); Carbohydrates: 2g; Fiber: 0g; Sugar: 1g; Sodium: 24mg; Protein: 1g

APPLE SAUCE

SERVES 12 / PREP TIME: 5 MINUTES / COOK TIME: 10 MINUTES

This apple sauce tastes delicious with pork, fish or dessert!

---

3 APPLES, PEELED AND CHOPPED

1 TBSP SKIM MILK OR EQUIVALENT

1/2 TSP NUTMEG

1/2 TSP CINNAMON

---

1. Steam the chopped apples over a steamer on a medium-high heat for 10 minutes.
2. Combine apples with the rest of the ingredients and blend in a food processor until smooth.
3. If you don't have a processor, cook for an extra 5 minutes and mash with a fork before passing through a sieve and adding the rest of the ingredients.
4. Serve right away or store in a sealable container in the fridge for 2-3 days.
5. Alternatively store in an ice cube tray and pop out to thaw before you need it.

Per serving: Calories: 36; Fat: 0g (Saturated Fat: 0g); Carbohydrates: 6.5g; Fiber: 1.25g; Sugar: 1.5g; Sodium: 0mg; Protein: 0g

DRINKS & DESSERTS

FRUIT SMOOTHIE

SERVES 2 / PREP TIME: 5 MINUTES / COOK TIME: N/A

Sooth symptoms with this healthy juice.

1/4 FROZEN SPINACH

1/4 CUP CANNED PINEAPPLE (UNSWEETENED), DICED

1 CUP SKIM MILK OR DAIRY FREE EQUIVALENT

---

1. Add all of the ingredients to a blender until smooth.
2. Serve cold over ice if desired!

Per serving: Calories: 52; Fat: 0g (Saturated Fat: 0g); Carbohydrates: 9g; Fiber: 0g; Sugar: 9g; Sodium: 55mg; Protein: 4g; Potassium: 251mg

HOMEMADE RICE MILK

SERVES 2 / PREP TIME: 5 MINUTES / COOK TIME: N/A

Use as a replacement for cow's milk.

---

1 CUP COOKED WHITE RICE

4 CUPS WATER

1/2 TSP STEVIA POWDER

1/2 TSP VANILLA EXTRACT

---

1. Add the ingredients to a blender or food processor for 5 minutes until smooth.
2. Strain through a sieve or muslin cloth to get rid of any bits.
3. Use right away or store in the fridge for 2-3 days.

Per serving: Calories: 105; Fat: 0g (Saturated Fat: 0g); Carbohydrates: 24g; Fiber: 0g; Sugar: 0g; Sodium: 1mg; Protein: 2g; Potassium: 29mg

STRAWBERRY MILKSHAKE

SERVES 2 / PREP TIME: 5 MINUTES / COOK TIME: N/A

Delicious fruit drink!

1/2 CUP CANNED STRAWBERRIES (UNSWEETENED)

2 TBSP FROZEN SPINACH

1 CUP SKIM MILK

1 TSP RAW HONEY

---

1. Blend all ingredients in a food processor until smooth and then strain through a sieve to remove seeds and pips.
2. Serve over ice.

Per serving: Calories: 73; Fat: 0g (Saturated Fat: 0g); Carbohydrates: 13g; Fiber: 2g; Sugar: 11g; Sodium: 76mg; Protein: 5g; Potassium: 327mg

NUTMEG & HONEY TREATS

SERVES 2 / PREP TIME: 15 MINUTES / COOK TIME: 15 MINUTES

Delicious sweet bites.

1/2 TSP STEVIA POWDER	1 TSP SUGAR
1/2 TSP GROUND NUTMEG	1/2 TSP SALT
1 SMALL EGG	1 TSP UNSALTED BUTTER
1/2 TBSP RAW HONEY	1 TSP WATER
2 TBSP SKIM MILK OR EQUIVALENT	
1/4 CUP WHITE FLOUR (GF IF NEEDED)	
1/2 TSP BAKING POWDER	

1. Preheat the oven to 375°f/190°c/Gas Mark 5.
2. Spray a baking sheet with cooking spray or lightly grease with butter.
3. Mix together stevia and nutmeg.
4. In a separate bowl mix together the egg, honey and milk.
5. In another bowl, mix the flour, baking powder, sugar, salt and butter.
6. Rub together with your fingers until a breadcrumb consistency is reached.
7. Add the milk mixture to the dry mixture and mix well.
8. Onto a lightly floured surface, roll out your dough with a rolling pin until roughly 5cm thick.
9. Brush with a little extra milk and dust with the nutmeg mixture from earlier.
10. Divide dough into 6 and roll into balls.
11. Add to the baking sheet, leaving at least 1inch gap between each dough ball.
12. Bake for 12-15 minutes or until your knife pulls out clean from the center.
13. Serve!

Per serving: Calories: 132; Fat: 4g (Saturated Fat: 2g); Carbohydrates: 21g; Fiber: 1g; Sugar: 7g; Sodium: 734mg; Protein: 4g; Potassium: 61mg

GRANDMA'S POACHED APPLES

SERVES 2 / PREP TIME: 5 MINUTES / COOK TIME: 25 MINUTES

Delicious!

---

2 SMALL APPLES, PEELED, CORED AND HALVED

2 CLOVES

1 TSP CINNAMON

1 TBSP FAT FREE GREEK YOGURT

---

1. Add the apples, cloves and cinnamon to a pot of water over a medium heat and simmer for 20-25 minutes or until apples are soft.
2. Serve hot with a helping of yogurt.

Per serving: Calories:35; Fat: 0g (Saturated Fat: 0g); Carbohydrates: 9g; Fiber: 2g; Sugar: 6g; Sodium: 4mg; Protein: 1g; Potassium:74mg

CONVERSION TABLES

Volume

Imperial	Metric
1 tbsp	15ml
2 fl oz	55 ml
3 fl oz	75 ml
5 fl oz (¼ pint)	150 ml
10 fl oz (½ pint)	275 ml
1 pint	570 ml
1 ¼ pints	725 ml
1 ¾ pints	1 liter
2 pints	1.2 liters
2½ pints	1.5 liters

Oven temperatures

Gas Mark	Fahrenheit	Celsius
1/4	225	110
1/2	250	130
1	275	140
2	300	150
3	325	170
4	350	180
5	375	190
6	400	200
7	425	220
8	450	230

Weight

Imperial	Metric
½ oz	10 g
¾ oz	20 g
1 oz	25 g
1½ oz	40 g
2 oz	50 g
2½ oz	60 g
3 oz	75 g
4 oz	110 g
4½ oz	125 g
5 oz	150 g
6 oz	175 g
7 oz	200 g
8 oz	225 g
9 oz	250 g
10 oz	275 g

BIBLIOGRAPHY

Olausson, E.A., Störsrud, S., Grundin, H., Isaksson, M., Attvall, S. and Simrén, M. (2014) 'A small particle size diet reduces upper gastrointestinal symptoms in patients with diabetic Gastroparesis: A Randomized controlled trial', The American Journal of Gastroenterology, 109(3), pp. 375–385. doi: 10.1038/ajg.2013.453. Garrick, R. (2008) 'Prevalence of chronic kidney disease in the United States', Yearbook of Medicine, 2008, pp. 215–217.

EMRAL, R. (2002) 'DIABETIC GASTROPARESIS (GASTROPARESIS DIABETICORUM)', Journal of Ankara Medical School, , pp. 001–008

PATRICK, A. and EPSTEIN, O. (2008) 'Review article: Gastroparesis', Alimentary Pharmacology & Therapeutics, 27(9), pp. 724–740.

Homko, C.J., Duffy, F., Friedenberg, F.K., Boden, G. and Parkman, H.P. (2015) 'Effect of dietary fat and food consistency on gastroparesis symptoms in patients with gastroparesis', Neurogastroenterology & Motility, 27(4), pp. 501–508

Nusrat, S. and Bielefeldt, K. (2012) 'Gastroparesis on the rise: Incidence vs awareness?', Neurogastroenterology & Motility, 25(1), pp. 16–22

Gastroparesis (2016) Available at: https://www.niddk.nih.gov/health-information/health-topics/digestive-diseases/gastroparesis/Pages/facts.aspx (Accessed: 6 September 2016).

American (2016) Gastroparesis. Available at: http://patients.gi.org/topics/gastroparesis/ (Accessed: 6 September 2016).

Staff, M.C. (2014) 'Gastroparesis definition', Mayoclinic, .

INDEX

Made in the USA
Columbia, SC
02 September 2022

66567013R00046